Guide To Survive Asthma

Asthma: Causes, Treatment, and Prevention - Healthline

By

Dr. Elliott Charles

Copyright ©2023 by Dr. Elliott Charles

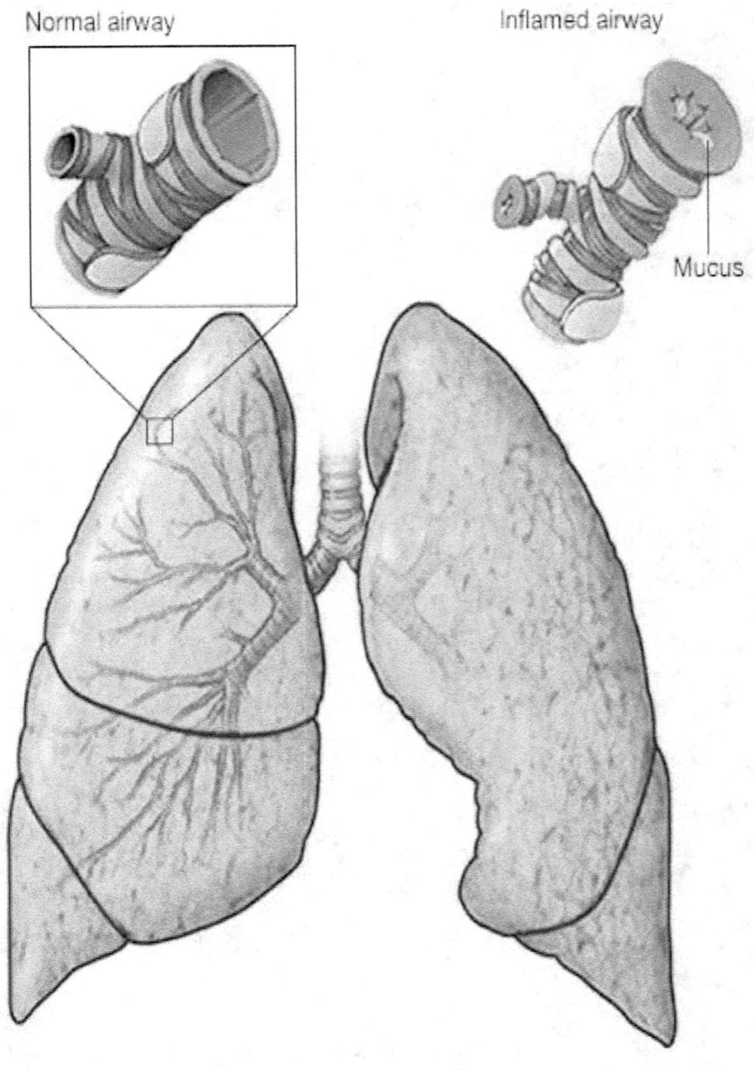
Normal airway
Inflamed airway
Mucus

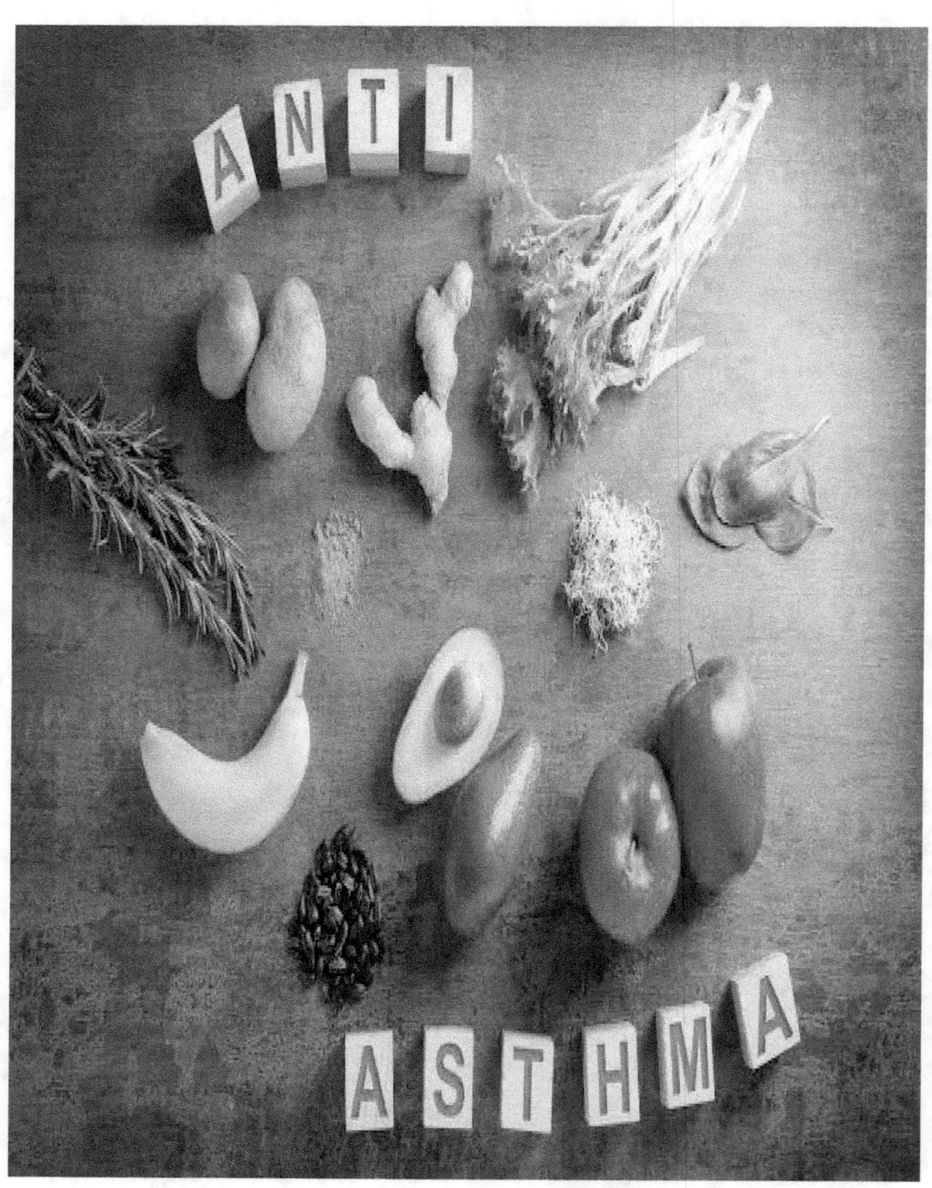
ANTI
ASTHMA

Table Of Contents

Introduction

The organs that are impacted by asthma are the lungs. One of the most prevalent chronic diseases affecting kids is asthma, while it can also affect adults. Asthma symptoms include coughing at night or in the early morning, wheezing, breathing difficulties, chest tightness, and wheezing. If you have asthma, you will always feel the effects of it; nevertheless, attacks only happen when something in your lungs is irritating.

Although there are many potential causes of asthma, we do know that occupational, environmental, and genetic variables have all been connected to the disorder.

If you have a close relative with asthma, your risk of developing the condition increases. Allergy-related asthma can be greatly influenced by a genetic propensity to develop atopy, an allergic condition. Allergic asthma is just one type of asthma, though.

Environmental elements including mold or moisture, dust mites and other allergens, as well as secondhand smoke, have been associated to asthma. Air pollution and viral lung infections can also cause asthma.

When a person who has never had asthma is exposed to anything at work, they can develop occupational asthma. This may occur if you develop an occupational allergy to something like mold or if you are frequently exposed to irritants like wood dust or chemicals at low levels or suddenly at high levels while working.

Particularly in young children under the age of five, asthma can be challenging to diagnose. A doctor's examination of your lungs and testing for allergens might reveal whether you have asthma.

During a checkup, a doctor will inquire if you frequently cough, particularly at night. He or she will also ask if your breathing problems are greater at particular seasons of the year or just after exercise. The doctor will then ask about chest pain, wheezing, and colds that linger longer than ten days after that. He or she will ask if anyone in your family currently has asthma, allergies, or any other respiratory conditions. Last but not least, the doctor will ask you about your house and see whether you've missed any work or school or if you have trouble performing specific activities.

The doctor might also conduct spirometry, a breathing test that gauges how much air you can exhale after taking a very deep breath both before and after taking asthma medication.

The signs of an asthma attack include coughing, chest tightness, wheezing, and trouble breathing. The attack occurs in the airways of your body, which transport air to your lungs. Your lungs' airways narrow as air passes through them,, like how the trunk of a tree is smaller than the branches. When you have asthma, the airways in your lungs enlarge on the sides and become narrower. Your body's natural production of mucus blocks your airways, limiting the amount of air that may enter and leave your lungs.

You can better control your disease by being aware of the warning symptoms of an asthma attack, avoiding triggers, and adhering to your doctor's recommendations. When asthma is in check:

You won't have to miss work or school, you won't cough or wheeze, you can still engage in all types of physical activity, and you won't need to go to the hospital. You'll also sleep better and experience less discomfort.

When "asthma triggers" are present in people with asthma, can an asthma attack happen?

An asthma attack might happen after exposure to "asthma triggers". The causes of your asthma may be very different from those of another individual. Find out what triggers you have and how to prevent them. Be alert for an assault if you are unable to evade your triggers. Some of the most frequent triggers include tobacco smoke, dust mites, outdoor air pollution, cockroach allergen, pets, mildew, smoke from burning wood or grass, and illnesses like the flu.

The Effects of Asthma on Your Body Your lungs always enlarge a little bit when you have asthma. The airways become more sensitive when they are exposed to viruses, allergies, irritants, or even emotions. Learn more about how the air we breathe affects our health.

Relapses in Asthma Your airways may enlarge significantly more and secrete more mucus during a flare-up. As a result, it is more challenging for air to enter and exit the lungs. The muscles that surround your airways might also contract, making breathing even more challenging. It is referred to as a "attack," "episode," or "flare-up" of asthma.

An asthma attack will undoubtedly leave you feeling exhausted. Moreover, a few days following an incident, you are more likely to have another flare-up. Ensure you: Within a few days of a flare-up:

Airway remodeling can be avoided by avoiding asthma triggers, monitoring your symptoms, or checking your airways with a peak flow meter. Inadequate asthma management or treatment might result in catastrophic problems including airway remodeling. Less air can pass through your airways as a result of lung scarring caused by asthma treatments losing their effectiveness. The airway does not need to be modified. To lessen asthma attacks, find a treatment strategy that works for you and see a health care provider. Take control of your asthma.

Chapter 1

Guide To Overcome Asthma

Information about asthma in numbers Low-income individuals, elderly individuals, Black, Hispanic, and Alaska Native people carry a disproportionate share of the burden of asthma in the United States. These demographics experience the highest incidence, hospitalizations, and deaths from asthma. Knowing about asthma Chronic asthma is characterized by airway edema and inflammation.

As a result, the airways that carry air from the mouth and nose to the lungs shorten.

Asthma symptoms include difficulty breathing (shortness of breath), wheezing, coughing, and tightness or pain in the chest.

Symptoms of asthma can have a variety of origins depending on the individual. Allergens like dust or cat dander are frequent causes of triggers. In certain people, exercise, stress, or exposure to cold air can potentially aggravate asthma symptoms.

A life-threatening and lethal condition is asthma.

Despite the fact that there is no known cure for asthma, the appropriate care can reduce your risk of episodes and enhance your quality of life.

Asthma is one of the most widespread and expensive diseases in the US. diseases.

How common is asthma?

Over 25 million people in the US suffer with asthma. In relation to 1 in 13 people, this. 1 Asthma affects over 20 million persons in the US who are 18 years of age or older. 1 The majority of Americans with adult asthma are black. 1 Asthma is more common in women than in males. Over 5.1 million children under the age of 18 suffer from asthma, which is a common chronic illness in youngsters. 1

Asthma is roughly three times as common in black children than in white kids. 1 Male children are more likely than female youngsters to have asthma.

How Often Do Kids Get Asthma Attacks?

Asthma affects approximately 8.4% of male children and 5.5% of female children.1

According to the Centers for Disease Control and Prevention (CDC), asthma attacks in children have decreased from 2001 to 2019.3 even though asthma is manageable, it is estimated that 50% of children with asthma have uncontrolled asthma.4

How Often Do Children Have Asthma Attacks?

Children with asthma who were 18 years old or younger reported having one or more attacks in 2019 at a rate of 44.3%. 1 Children with asthma under the age of five reported having an attack in about 47.2% of cases. 1

40.4% of persons with asthma who were 18 years of age or older reported having one or more attacks in 2018.

1 In America, adults of color experience more asthma attacks than any other group. 1 According to the CDC, fewer adult asthma attacks occurred between 2001 and 2019. 3

In 2018, 5.8 million visits to the doctor's office were related to asthma. 5 In addition, asthma accounted for 1.6 million visits to the emergency room and 178,530 discharges from hospital inpatient care in 2018. 6 Asthma-related visits to the emergency room are roughly five times as common among black Americans than white Americans in the United States.

How Many Asthma Deaths Take Place?

Each day, asthma results in the deaths of 11 Americans. Asthma caused the deaths of 4,145 people in 2020. With the appropriate treatment and care, nearly all of these deaths can be avoided. 8 In 2020, asthma-related deaths increased for the first time in twenty years. Black people in the United States are nearly three times more likely to die from asthma than white people in the United States.8 When sex is taken into account, Black females have the highest rate of asthma fatalities.8 Female adults are five times more likely to die from asthma than male adults, and male children are more likely to die from asthma than female children.8

What frequently causes asthma attacks?

By 2020, the risk of dying from asthma was nearly four times higher in Black women than in White men.

If you come into contact with irritants, you could experience an asthma attack. The term "triggers" for these substances is used by healthcare professionals. Knowing what triggers asthma episodes makes it simpler to prevent them.

For some people, a trigger can spark an attack right away. Attacks might start hours, days, or even years after they happen for other people or at other times.

Triggers can differ for each individual. Nonetheless, a few frequent triggers are as follows:

Polluted air: An asthma attack can be triggered by many things outside. Emissions from factories, car exhaust, smoke from wildfires, and more all contribute to air pollution.

Mildew mites: Even though you can't see them, these bugs are in our homes. This could trigger an asthma attack if you have an allergy to dust mites.

Exercise: Exercising can cause an attack for some people.

Mold: Mold can grow in damp places, which can be problematic for asthmatics. Even if you're not allergic to mold, you can have an attack.

Posts: Asthma attacks can be triggered by household pests like cockroaches and mice.

Pets: Asthma attacks can be triggered by pets. Inhaling pet dander, also known as dried skin flakes, can irritate your airways if you have an allergy.

Cigarette smoke: You are more likely to develop asthma if you or someone in your home smokes. Smoking should never be done in enclosed spaces like a car or home, and quitting is the best option. Your service provider can help.

Strong odors or chemicals. Some people may suffer attacks as a result of these things.

certain exposures in the workplace. At your job, you might come into contact with cleaning products, flour or wood dust, or other chemicals. If you have asthma, any one of these could be a trigger.

Everyone can develop asthma.

At any age, anyone can develop asthma. People with allergies or those who are exposed to cigarette smoke are more likely to develop asthma. This covers secondhand smoke as well as thirdhand smoke, which is when someone is exposed to clothing or surfaces after smoking (exposure to someone else who is smoking).

Asthma is more prevalent in girls than males born to these genders, according to statistics. Asthma is more prevalent among black people than other racial groups.

Why do men and women have different asthma prevalence rates?

Children who suffer from asthma are more likely to be male than female. In adulthood, female adults are more likely than male adults to have asthma.11 According to some studies, this trend reverses because testosterone affects lung cells. It has been discovered that the male sex hormone testosterone can lessen the swelling of the airways in asthma.11

Chapter 2

Symptoms, Causes, and Therapy for Asthma

Experts are unsure of the reasons why some people have asthma and others do not. Yet additional factors heighten the risk:

Allergies: Asthma is more prone to develop in people who have allergies.

environmental elements: Asthma can develop as a result of airway irritation. Among these chemicals include allergens, poisons, gases, and second- or third-hand smoke. They are especially dangerous to babies and young children whose immune systems are still growing.

Genetics: If you have a family history of asthma or an allergic condition, you are more likely to develop it.

Infections of the lungs: The developing lungs of young children can be harmed by certain respiratory infections, such as a respiratory syncytial virus (RSV).

What kind of asthma are there?

Based on the kind of the condition and the intensity of the symptoms, there are numerous categories into which asthma can be subdivided. Asthma, according to medical professionals, is:

You can feel normal in between attacks because this type of asthma comes and goes.

persistent: If you have asthma, your attacks generally happen frequently. How often you experience symptoms will determine how severe your asthma is. They also take your ability to react swiftly to an attack into account.

The following are some of the root causes of asthma:

Some people's asthma attacks are brought on by allergies. Examples of allergies include pet dander, pollen, and mold.

Non-allergic: Environmental variables may aggravate asthma. Exercise, stress, illness, or the environment all have the potential to trigger flare-ups.

Asthma can also be:

Adult-onset asthma: After the age of 18, this kind of asthma starts to appear.

Pediatric: This kind of asthma, often known as childhood asthma, can affect infants and young children and usually starts before the age of five. Children with asthma may outgrow it. Make sure to discuss this with your doctor before choosing whether your child needs an inhaler in case they experience an asthma attack. The physician who treats your kid can give you further details about the hazards.

The following types of asthma are also present:

Asthma brought on by exercise: Exercise is what causes this type, which is also known as exercise-induced bronchospasm.

Asthma in the workplace: Most people who work around irritating substances suffer from this kind of asthma.

ACOS: Asthma-COPD overlap syndrome When you have both asthma and chronic obstructive pulmonary disease (COPD), this type occurs. Breathing becomes difficult with either disease.

What signs and symptoms of asthma are there?

Asthma sufferers typically exhibit obvious symptoms. These signs are reminiscent of those seen with other respiratory infections:

sneezing chest pressure, pain, or tightening (particularly at night).

breathing problems

Wheezing.

Some of these symptoms may not be present when your asthma attacks. Different signs and symptoms of chronic asthma can appear at different times. Symptoms of asthma might also alter between attacks.

What triggers the majority of asthma attacks?

An asthma attack could occur if you come into contact with irritants. These substances are known as "triggers" by healthcare providers. It's easier to avoid asthma attacks when you know what causes them.

A trigger can immediately start an attack for some people. An attack may begin hours or days after it occurs for other people or at other times.

Each person's triggers may differ. However, some typical triggers include:

Polluted air: An asthma attack can be triggered by many things outside. Emissions from factories, car exhaust, smoke from wildfires, and more all contribute to air pollution.

Mildew mites: Even though you can't see them, these bugs are in our homes. This could trigger an asthma attack if you have an allergy to dust mites.

Exercise: Exercising can cause an attack for some people.

Mold: Mold can grow in damp places, which can be problematic for asthmatics. Even if you're not allergic to mold, you can have an attack.

Posts: Asthma attacks can be triggered by household pests like cockroaches and mice.

Pets: Asthma attacks can be triggered by pets. Inhaling pet dander, also known as dried skin flakes, can irritate your airways if you have an allergy.

Cigarette smoke: You are more likely to develop asthma if you or someone in your home smokes. Smoking should never be done in enclosed spaces like a car or home, and quitting is the best option. Your service provider can help.

Strong odors or chemicals. Some people may suffer attacks as a result of these things.

certain exposures in the workplace. At your job, you might come into contact with cleaning products, flour or wood dust, or other chemicals. If you have asthma, any one of these could be a trigger.

An asthma attack is what?

Your airways' muscles are relaxed while you breathe regularly, allowing air to move freely and softly. During an asthma episode, three things can happen: Bronchospasm: Tightening of the muscles surrounding the airways (constrict). Your airways become smaller when you get tight. A restricted airway prevents air from moving freely.

The lining of your airways swells because of inflammation. Your lungs are unable to take in as much air when your airways are inflamed. Mucus production: During an assault, your body produces more mucus. The airways are blocked by the thick mucus.

When you breathe out, wheezing is the sound your airways make because they become more clogged. Exacerbation or flare-up are other terms for an asthma episode. It describes a situation in which it is impossible to regulate your asthma.

How is asthma identified by medical experts?
Your healthcare professional will examine your medical history, which will include details about your parents and siblings. Your healthcare professional will also ask you about your symptoms. Your doctor is going to want to know if you've ever had allergies, eczema, which is an itchy rash caused by allergies, or any other lung conditions.
.Your physician might recommend spirometry. By measuring the airflow through your lungs, this test is used to diagnose you and monitor your recovery. A skin test, blood test, or chest X-ray might be ordered by your doctor.

Chapter 3

Scientific approved Treatment for Asthma

There are options for managing your asthma. Your doctor may recommend medication to reduce symptoms. Some examples are:

The muscles that surround your airways are relaxed by bronchodilators. Because the muscles are relaxed, the airways can move air. They also make it easier for mucus to pass through the airways. These drugs are used to treat symptoms as they appear in both intermittent and chronic asthma.

Drugs that lower inflammation includes: These drugs lessen the mucus production and swelling in your airways. They make breathing in and out of your lungs easier. Your doctor may have prescribed them for daily use to treat or avoid the symptoms of your persistent asthma.

Asthma biologic treatments: When proper inhaler therapy fails to alleviate severe asthma symptoms, these are the medications of choice.

Asthma medications can be taken in a variety of ways. The drugs can be inhaled via a nebulizer, metered-dose inhaler, or another kind of asthma inhaler. Your doctor might prescribe oral drugs for you to take.

What is the management of asthma?

The goal of asthma treatment is to lessen symptoms. Controlling your asthma means:

at work and at home to do as you choose.

possess hardly any or no asthma symptoms.

Use your rescue inhaler (relief medication) sparingly.

Sleep disruption occurs even if you don't have asthma.

What is the asthma treatment?

It's critical to keep an eye on your asthma symptoms. The management of diseases depends on it. A peak flow (PF) meter can be requested from your healthcare provider. This device controls how quickly you can expel air from your lungs. That could assist your doctor in adjusting your medication. Also, it reveals whether your symptoms are getting worse.

How can asthma symptoms be tracked?

Even if you have asthma, you can still get a lot done and enjoy sports and other activities. Manage your symptoms, discover your triggers, and prevent or manage attacks with the assistance of your healthcare provider.

What is the outlook for someone who has asthma?

An asthma action plan will be developed together with you by your healthcare provider. How and when to take your medications are outlined in this plan. It also tells you when to get emergency care and what to do based on your asthma symptoms. If you have any questions, you should talk to your doctor.

Speak with your doctor if you have any inquiries right away or if you have a severe asthma attack.

What must I do in the event of a serious asthma attack?

Make use of your rescue inhaler as soon as possible. Your airways are opened by medicines that work quickly in a rescue inhaler. It is not the same as a daily-use maintenance inhaler. The rescue inhaler should be used when symptoms are bothering you, and if your flare is severe, you can use it more frequently.

If you don't have a rescue inhaler with you or it doesn't work, go to the emergency room.

Panic or anxiety

Fingernails and lips that are bluish (in people with light skin tones) or gray or whitish (in people with dark skin tones)

Pressure or pain in the chest

wheezing when you breathe or persistent coughing.

Trouble speaking.

a pale, sweaty face.

Breathing very quickly or rapidly

How can you tell if you have asthma or not?

A doctor must be seen to ascertain whether you have asthma or another ailment. Other respiratory issues may make it difficult to breathe or result in coughing and wheezing.

Nighttime asthma or nocturnal asthma are terms used to describe asthma that gets worse at night. Although there are some educated guesses as to why this occurs, there are no established causes. These are some:

Why is my asthma worse at night?

How you go to bed: Sleeping on your back can cause acid reflux or mucus to return to your stomach from your throat. Additionally, sleeping on your back puts pressure on your lungs and chest, making it harder to breathe. On the other hand, lying on your side or face down can put pressure on your lungs.

Things that happen in the evening and your bedroom: Your pillows, sheets, and blankets may have mold, dust mites, or pet hair on them. You might have brought pollen inside if you were outside in the early evening.

Effects of the medication: Steroids and montelukast, two asthma medications, can disrupt your sleep.

Air that is either too hot or cold: When you breathe in hot air, narrowing of the airways can occur. Some people get asthma when they breathe in cold air.

Changes in lung function: As a natural process, nighttime lung function declines.

During the day, asthma is poorly controlled: When not managed during the day, symptoms will not improve at night. Working with your doctor to control your asthma symptoms throughout the day and night is essential. It's critical to treat symptoms at night. Nighttime asthma attacks can be deadly and even fatal.

What should I understand about COVID-19 and asthma?

If you get COVID-19, you are more likely to need to be hospitalized if you have moderate-to-severe asthma or if your asthma symptoms are not well controlled. As a result, if you go indoors with others, you should wear a mask, get vaccinated, and stay away from people who have the virus.

Chapter 4

Reverse And reducing the risk of ASTHMA in the future

Keeping an ASTHMA Recurrent Risk at Bay If you have asthma, you should do all in your power to limit your exposure to asthma triggers. Understanding what causes you to cough, wheeze, and struggle to breathe is the first step. Although there is no known treatment for asthma, there are steps you may take to manage it and stop attacks.

1. Identify Asthma Triggers Some asthma triggers can cause a series of symptoms to appear. These are some:
Polluting the air
Allergies Cold air A virus like the flu or cold Exercise Sinusitis Smoking Fragrances It's important to know your asthma triggers and how to avoid them.

For several weeks, keep track of your symptoms in an asthma diary. Describe in detail all of the emotional and environmental factors that cause your asthma. Check your diary whenever you have an asthma attack to see what, if anything, might have caused it. Molds and cockroaches, two common asthma triggers, are not always obvious. Tests to identify the allergens you react to should be discussed with your asthma specialist. Then take preventative measures.
Take precautions to avoid having an asthma attack if you are planning a strenuous workout, have asthma that is caused by exercise, or plan to exercise in the cold, dry, or humid air. Follow your doctor's

instructions for treating asthma, which typically includes using an albuterol-containing asthma inhaler before exercising.

2 Avoid Allergens If you suffer from asthma or allergies, it is essential to avoid allergens (things to which you are allergic). Exposure to allergens can temporarily increase airway inflammation, increasing the likelihood of an attack.

3. Smoking of any kind is a bad combination for asthma. Reduce your reliance on tobacco, incense, candles, fires, and fireworks as smoke sources. Avoid public areas where smoking is permitted and do not permit it in your home or vehicle. If you smoke, seek assistance in quitting. Asthma is always made worse by smoking.

4. Do what you can to stay healthy to prevent colds. Because contracting a cold or the flu will exacerbate your asthma symptoms, avoid close contact. If you handle anything that a person with a respiratory infection may have touched, thoroughly wash your hands.

5. Reduce the likelihood of having an asthma attack by allergen-proofing your home, whether you're at home, at work, or on the road. There are steps you can take to make your home allergy-proof. Never eat at a restaurant that smokes or allows smoking. Choose a hotel room without smoking. Bring your pillows and bedding if you can, in case the hotel only has down comforters and feather pillows. Asthma symptoms can be brought on by dust mites housed in them.

6. Get Vaccinated Every year, get vaccinated against the flu, which can make your asthma worse for days or weeks. You are more likely to be hospitalized as a result of flu complications like pneumonia if you have asthma. Neuromas, a vaccine against pneumonia, should be given to anyone over the age of 19 every 5 to 10 years. Additionally, you are more likely to contract pneumococcal pneumonia, a common form of bacterial pneumonia. In addition, you need the Tap and zoster vaccines to avoid shingles and protect yourself from tetanus, diphtheria, and whooping cough.

7. If your doctor finds that you have allergies, allergy shots (immunotherapy) may help keep your

asthma from getting worse and allergy symptoms from coming back. The doctor injects small amounts of the allergen under your skin regularly with allergy shots. Your body may become accustomed to the allergen over time and react less to being exposed to it. Keep your asthma under control with this.

8. Asthma medications that are prescribed for a long time are meant to stop symptoms and attacks. Even if you don't experience any symptoms, you still need to take them every day. They will reduce inflammation in your airways and maintain asthma control, reducing the likelihood of a flare-up. Talk to your doctor about switching to a different treatment if side effects bother you.

9. Follow Your Asthma Action Plan: Even when you feel fine, take your medication. Always have an inhaler on you. Check your treatment plan for medication dosage instructions if you notice symptoms. The plan can tell you when to call a doctor and what medications will help during an attack.

10. Make use of a home peak flow meter to see how well the air moving through your lungs is moving. Your airways narrow when you are attacked. Before you experience any symptoms, the meter can alert you to this happening hours or days in advance. This gives you time to take the prescribed medications and possibly stop the attack before it begins.

How Can I Prevent Infections That Trigger Asthma?

You can help prevent infections that can cause asthma symptoms by doing the following:

Get your hands clean. Maintaining good hygiene can lower your risk of contracting viral infections like the flu. To get rid of germs that remain on your hands, remember to wash them frequently throughout the day.

Get vaccinated. If you want to get the flu shot every year, talk to your doctor. In addition, talk about the possibility of getting vaccinated against pneumococcal pneumonia. Pneumococcus is a common bacteria that can cause bacterial pneumonia, which can be especially bad for asthmatics.

Keep sinusitis at bay. To assist in preventing asthma attacks, be aware of the symptoms of a sinus infection and notify your doctor as soon as possible.
Asthma medication and equipment should not be shared. You should not share your nebulizer, mouthpiece, nebulizer tubing, or asthma inhaler with anybody.
What kinds of flu shots are there?
There are two types of flu vaccine: a shot and a spray for the nose.

What Types of Flu Vaccines Are Available
There is no live virus in flu shots, so they cannot cause the flu. FluMist, a vaccine for the nasal flu, does not contain flu viruses that have been weakened. The flu shot, not FluMist, should be given to asthmatics.

Some other choices include:
Smaller needles are used for intradermal injections, and they only penetrate the top layer of the skin rather than the muscle. They are for people between the ages of 18 and 64.
For individuals between the ages of 18 and 49 who suffer from severe egg allergies, egg-free vaccines are now available.

For those over 65, high-dose vaccines may be more effective in preventing the flu.

How Do Flu Vaccines Work in People With Asthma?

Everyone receives the flu vaccine in the same way, including asthmatics. Your body develops antibodies as a result of them. The flu is prevented from spreading by these antibodies. Some people may experience muscle aches and fatigue as a result of this antibody reaction.

The flu vaccine contains a variety of flu viruses every year. The strains that were selected are those that, according to researchers, are most likely to appear that year. The flu vaccine is about 60% effective at preventing the flu if the choice is made correctly. However, people who are older or have a weaker immune system are less likely to benefit from the vaccine.

Who should receive a flu shot?

Every year, everyone over the age of six months should get the flu shot, according to the CDC. The flu vaccine is particularly important for many groups. Either they themselves are more susceptible to flu-related complications or they are in close proximity to others who are. These are some:

Adults and children with chronic health conditions, such as asthma and other conditions that depress the immune system; caregivers for those at risk for flu-related complications, such as health care workers and caregivers to very young children; Older people who live in nursing homes and other long-term care facilities. When should asthmatics get their flu shots?

The flu shot is best received as soon as it becomes available, ideally by October, if you have asthma. The flu season can start as early as October and continue through May. But if the flu virus is still present, getting vaccinated in January or later can be beneficial. The flu vaccine takes about two weeks to become fully effective at preventing the flu.

Where can I get an influenza shot?

The American Lung Association offers an automated clinic finder for the flu shot (ALA). Visit the organization's website, input your zip code, and choose one or more dates to learn about forthcoming clinics in your neighborhood. You can also ask your pharmacist for advice. Most retail pharmacies sell the flu vaccination.

Adult Asthma Control

Effective asthma management involves these five steps:

1. Stay on top of your symptoms by adhering to an asthma action plan. By adhering to an asthma action plan, you are better able to manage your symptoms and reduce your risk of spending time in the hospital with asthma.

All of the information you need is in one place in an asthma action plan. Every day, it teaches you how to take care of your asthma. Additionally, it explains what to do if your asthma worsens.

Download an action plan if you haven't already, and make an appointment to see your doctor or asthma nurse so they can complete it with you.

2. Even if you are feeling well, take your preventer every day. Over time, the medicine builds up protection. It prevents inflammation of your

airways, making you less likely to react to your triggers.

Your risk of developing symptoms and having an asthma attack will be reduced if you adhere to a good routine and take your medication as directed.

It could mean that you don't have any symptoms at all, allowing you to continue with your life without having to worry about asthma getting in the way.

3. Always carry your reliever inhaler with you wherever you go so that you can quickly treat any unforeseen symptoms.

You can use your action plan to identify any signs that your asthma is getting worse. An asthma attack can be avoided if you act quickly.

If you use your reliever inhaler at least three times per week, it's a sign that your asthma is getting worse, and you should see a doctor or an asthma nurse right away.

4. Check how you use your inhaler There are so many different kinds of inhalers that it can be hard to know how to use one.

How much medicine gets into your airways where it's needed depends a lot on how you use your inhaler. You should notice fewer symptoms if you do it right.

If you take your inhaler correctly, you can also help prevent side effects from the medication remaining in your mouth.

You can see how to use a variety of inhalers and spacers in action right now because we have instructional videos available. Also, every time you get your asthma review, ask your doctor or asthma nurse to check it for you.

5. Perform an annual asthma review A once-a-year asthma review is a chance to review your inhaler technique and update your asthma action plan.

To keep your symptoms under control, you can make sure you are taking the right medications at the right times.

Even if you're doing well with your asthma, it's still worth going so you can make sure you're still doing everything you can to avoid having an asthma attack.

"If your symptoms worsen or if you use your Jreliever inhaler more than three times per week, schedule an additional appointment so you can be evaluated. can get more support in keeping your asthma under control,"

Managing Asthma In Teens

Managing Asthma in Teens: Ways to Breathe Better Recognize your strategy. Ask your doctor to explain the significance of each action plan step and medication. You'll feel more in charge if you know exactly what is going on. When you see your doctor, go over the plan and explain where you might have struggled with it.

Utilize tools for managing asthma. If daily long-term control medications, also known as "controller" or "maintenance" medications, are a part of your treatment plan, don't stop taking them even if you're feeling fine. Although it can be tempting to only take occasional quick-relief medications and skip the recommended daily medications, this typically does not work.

Establish a schedule. It's easy to forget to take your medication, but if you plan to do other asthma management tasks and take your medications at the same time every day, this is less likely to happen. Like brushing your teeth, and taking your medication in your daily routine.

Avoid smoking. If you smoke, talk to your parent or a doctor about how to stop. Don't stand next to your friends who smoke because secondhand smoke is a common cause of asthma attacks. Talk to someone in your family who smokes about quitting.

Take charge of the environment. If you have asthma, environmental triggers like pet dander and dust mites can be harmful. Keep Fido and Fluffy out of your bedroom if you have pets. Also, try to keep the dust out of your room by cleaning it often and talking to your doctor about using special pillows and mattress covers.

Every year, get a flu shot. Health officials advise that all children and adolescents receive flu shots. For asthmatics, flu shots are especially important. A person with asthma who gets the flu has a greater chance of getting a more severe illness.

Choose a sport or activity that suits your schedule. Swimming and baseball, for example, are less likely to cause asthma attacks. However, many athletes have discovered that any sport, even endurance or cold-weather sports, can be played with the right training and medication. Sports can improve your mood, which is helpful when you're feeling frustrated about having asthma.

Managing asthma with a management plan is beneficial for more than just your health. You can develop the discipline to stick to a plan and succeed in other areas of your life by getting used to following an asthma action plan.

Your Daily Guide to Managing Asthma Well.

Chronic asthma is a condition; People who have it will have to deal with it for the rest of their lives. If you or someone you care about is one of the estimated 25 million Americans with asthma, you know how important it is to stay on top of the condition by learning more about what causes your symptoms and how to avoid flare-ups.

Handling Asthma Complications and Everyday Life

Asthma Management and Its Complications There is no one-size-fits-all approach to asthma management. Asthma can be a minor inconvenience for some people; It can be a serious, even life-threatening condition for some people. Some people may only experience asthma symptoms on occasion in response to particular triggers, while others may experience symptoms on a regular basis that are severe enough to make it difficult to go about their daily lives. Additionally, there are a variety of asthma types, including allergy-induced asthma and exercise-induced bronchoconstriction (EIB), which is asthma that is brought on by physical exertion.

Chapter 5

Alternatives for Treating Asthma Using Natural and Homeopathic Items

The use of natural products for the treatment of physiologic disorders, particularly when combined with other drugs, has been widely reported in ethno pharmacological studies as an important scientific tool for bioprospecting exploration and the discovery of new bioactive compounds from natural sources. Natural products can also be used to treat asthma. Drugs derived from natural sources still make a significant contribution to the discovery and development of new medicines despite the extensive scientific progress that has been made in chemical and pharmaceutical technology regarding the process of synthesizing new molecules. In the beginning, these studies are based on the traditional use of natural products. These products are popular with pharmaceutical companies because they are cheap and easy to use, making it possible for them to conduct numerous studies on their therapeutic properties, toxicity, and safety.

In addition, a significant alternative for the treatment of a number of diseases is the utilization of natural products as complementary therapies. About 40% of conventional treatments in the United States of America are supplemented with natural products, vitamins, and other dietary supplements. Natural products are used to treat a variety of illnesses, including allergic and inflammatory conditions. Since the Chinese culture employed the infusion of Ephedra sinica, which is an immune system stimulator able to reduce asthma crises, traditional medicine has documented the use of plant-based medicines for the treatment of asthma for over 5000 years In fact, the alternative medicine literature indicates that the use of these products is associated with biochemical mechanisms involved in immunomodulation, which could contribute to the management of these diseases. A more recent study by Costa and colleagues described the primary natural sources that Brazilian families in the Northeast Region of the country used to treat asthma. Beet, honey, onion, garlic, yarrow, and mint were all included in the study, demonstrating the wide range of natural products used to treat asthma in children. In addition, natural oils from plants and animals, which can be obtained through a variety of extraction methods, have been cited a lot in the treatment of asthma. Because of the presence of compounds like phenylpropanoids and mono- and sesquiterpenes as the primary bioactive compounds that provide their anti-inflammatory, antifungal, antibacterial, and anesthetic properties, plant-derived natural oils are the primary natural products used in the complementary asthma therapy In a similar vein, animal-derived oils have been utilized. They contain a variety of saturated, monounsaturated, and polyunsaturated fatty acids, as well as compounds from animal organs and secretions that regulate tissue oxidative capacity and immune modulation. Bioactive compounds that are capable of inhibiting COX-2 and COX-5 are linked to the activity attributed to oils derived from animals and plants. By lowering the levels of IL-4, IL-5, and IL-13 cytokines, reducing the activity and proliferation of NK cells, increasing the level of endogenous corticosteroids, contributing to the regulation of the NF-B pathway, and reducing the production of mucus and inflammation in lung tissues, these compounds can also alter the function of immune cells displays all of the products that were discovered in the studies that were included in this review after the inclusion criteria were evaluated. This review only describes plant-derived products with three or more citations because of their wide range of them. On the other hand, because there aren't many scientific studies on the anti-inflammatory properties of natural products derived from animals and microorganisms, the following sections describe all studies that met the inclusion criteria.

Natural Asthma Treatment using Plant-Based Products

Natural Products Obtained from Plants for Rapid Asthma Treatment The use of natural products derived from plants in traditional medicine has been documented for centuries, particularly in China, Japan, and India. As a result, the topics that follow focus on these products or bioactive compounds derived from the most researched plants that are utilized in asthma treatment.

Flavonoids

The presence of two benzene rings (A and B) linked by a heterocyclic pyrene ring (C) is the chemical characteristic of flavonoids, which come from plants, nuts, and fruits. They are one of many polyphenolic secondary metabolites, of which over 8,000 distinct compounds have already been identified. They are categorized as flavans, flavanones, isoflavonoids, flavones, isoflavones, anthocyanidins, and flavonolignans based on their chemical structure. Flavans or isoflavones contain chromane, a heterocyclic hydrocarbon skeleton, and a phenyl group (B ring) is added to its carbon 2 or 3 C ring. An oxo-group is present in position 4 for the flavanones and isoflavones. Flavones and isoflavones are identified by the double bonds between C2 and C3, and anthocyanidins are identified by the double bonds between C1 and C2 Their wide range of physiological and biological activities is facilitated by their diverse chemical structures, which include antioxidant, anti-inflammatory, antiallergic, antiviral, hepatoprotective, antithrombotic, and anticarcinogenic properties 14 studies included in this review identified flavonoids as a class of compounds that could be used to treat asthma. The primary flavonoids with an antiasthmatic activity that have been reported in the literature and are utilized in traditional medicine are outlined in the sections that follow. According to these studies, the phytocomplex's presence played a role in the antiasthmatic activity of plant extracts containing these compounds.

(1) Compounds of flavones: Oroxylin A, Baicalin, Luteolin, and Chrysin. Chrysin, which is defined as 5,7-dihydroxy-2-phenyl-1-4H-chromene-4-one, is a flavone that can be found in propolis and other plants. It is also present in the flowers of Passiflora incarnata and Passiflora caerulea. Chrysin is a substance that suppresses the proliferation of airway smooth muscle cells and promotes a decrease in the levels of interferon-, IL-4, IL-13, IgE, and interferon-, both of which reduce the asthma inflammatory process. Bae and co. used an in vitro cell culture model to describe the chrysin's ability to promote the inhibition of proinflammatory cytokines in their research. Since calcium is necessary for the transcription of proinflammatory cytokine genes, they suggested that the reduction of intracellular calcium in mast cells was the cause of this effect

[90]. In addition, Yao and colleagues' investigation of the asthma-fighting capacity of chrysin in mice sensitized to ovalbumin (OVA) Chrysin appeared to be a promising compound that could be used to control asthmatic clinical signs and remodeling of the airways

Baicalin is a natural metabolite that can be easily found in the leaves and barks of several species of the Scutellaria genus. It is a 7-glucuronic acid-5,6-dihydroxyflavone. Using an asthma-induced animal model, Park and colleagues investigated baicalin's anti-inflammatory activity. The bronchoalveolar lavage fluids (BALF) showed that this compound reduced inflammatory cell infiltration and TNF-levels. The activity of baicalin was credited with the fact that this metabolite decreases the TNF expression induced by lipopolysaccharides on macrophages and selectively inhibits the enzyme activity of PDE4 suggesting that this metabolite could be utilized in the treatment of asthma.

Moreover, luteolin
Additionally, aromatic flowering plants like Salvia tomentose and Lamiaceae, as well as broccoli, green pepper, parsley, and thyme, contain luteolin (2-(3,4-

dihydroxy phenyl)-5,7-dihydroxy-4-chromone), which has also been shown to be effective against asthma. Through inhibition of the GABAergic system, which is responsible for the excessive production of mucus during the asthmatic crisis as a result of overstimulation of the epithelial cells, Shen and colleagues investigated its pharmacological activity. By partially inhibiting GABA activities, this compound was found to be able to reduce goblet cell hyperplasia, according to the study

Oroxylin A, a flavone found in the extract of Oroxylum indicum tree and Scutellaria baicalensis Georgi, is another antiasthmatic flavonoid compound. Oroxylin A, or 5-7-dihydroxy-6-methoxy-2-phenylchromen-4-one, was able to reduce the levels of IL-4, IL-5, IL-13, and OVA-specific IgE in BALF, as well as the airway hyperactivity in an OVA-induced asthma murine model, as stated by Zhou. Oroxylin A's ability to prevent inflammatory cell infiltration in the perivascular and peribronchial areas, as determined by histopathological examination, was also demonstrated in this study.

(2) Compounds of flavonoids: Kaempferol, galanin, and quercetin. Quercetin (2-(3,4-dihydroxy phenyl)-

3,5,7-trihydroxy-4H-chrome-4-one), a flavonol compound that is found in a lot of onions, apples, broccoli, cereals, grapes, tea, and wine, is known to be the main active compound of these plants. Because of this, these plants are used a lot in traditional medicine to treat inflammatory, allergic, and viral diseases. As in vitro and in vivo models, cell cultures and rats were used in this compound's anti-asthma research, demonstrating its strong ability to reduce inflammatory processes. These studies suggest that quercetin works by inhibiting lipoxygenase and PDE4 and reducing histamine and leukotriene release, which in turn reduces the formation of proinflammatory cytokines and the production of IL-4, respectively. Quercetin also inhibited human mast cell activation by inhibiting prostaglandin release and inhibiting Ca2+ influx favoring the therapeutic relief of asthma symptoms and decreasing the dependence on short-acting - agonists.

Using a specific-pathogen-free mouse model, Galangin, a chemically defined compound known as 3,5,7-trihydroxy-2-phenylchromen-4-one, was evaluated for its pharmacological activity Galangin is readily available on Alpinia officinarum Liu's study demonstrated a reduction in ROS levels in vitro and an effective response to OVA-induced inflammation in vivo. In addition, galanin inhibited goblet cell hyperplasia, decreased TGF-1 levels, and inhibited the expression of vascular endothelial grown factor (VEGF) and matrix metalloproteinase-9 (MMP-9) in BEHALF or lung tissue, making it an asthmatic anti remodeling agent. Its anti-remodeling activity in the TGF-1-ROS-MAPK pathway was highlighted by this result, demonstrating its potential for asthma treatment

Kaempferol, also known as 3,5,7-trihydroxy-2-(4-hydroxyphenyl)-4H-chromed-4-one, is a flavonol that can be found in a variety of plant sources, including apples, broccoli, and citrus fruits Due to its pharmacological potential, particularly against inflammation, this substance has been studied. Chung et al.'s study found that a mouse model of asthma with OVA-induced airway inflammation was used to demonstrate that kaempferol can significantly reduce the inflammatory process by reducing the production of inflammatory cytokines and IgE antibodies and the infiltration of inflammatory cells. In addition, the airway inflammation reaction's intracellular ROS production was reduced by this compound

In addition, Mahat et al. demonstrated that kaempferol inhibits nitric oxide and inhibits nitric oxide-induced COX-2 enzyme activation, further reducing prostaglandin-E2 production and inhibiting the cytotoxic effects of nitric oxide.

The previously mentioned Chung this book also describes the antiasthma activity of kaempferol-3-O-rhamnoside, a glycosylated derivative of kaempferol, to increase the likelihood of using kaempferol as a bioactive in the development of new drugs or medicines. The glycosylation of kaempferol made it more soluble and stable, as well as less toxic. This made it possible to make a compound that has a lot of potentials to help asthma patients. This justification suggests that the anti-inflammatory properties of plant extracts that contain this substance and have been used to treat asthma may be due to the presence of this compound.

Resveratrol

Resveratrol is a natural stilbenoid compound that comes from the bark of red fruits. It is a class of polyphenols that are known to be antioxidant and has promising anti-inflammatory and asthmatic properties. Hu et al. used eosinophils from asthmatics in their research and demonstrated that resveratrol induces not only cell cycle arrest in the G1/S phase but also apoptosis, resulting in a decrease in the number of eosinophils and, consequently, the prevention of histamine and PGD-2 release, bronchoconstriction, vasodilatation, and mucus production (Figure 1). In addition, Lee and colleagues demonstrated that resveratrol was effective against the asthmatic mouse model by reducing the plasma concentration of T-helper-2-type cytokines like IL-4 and IL-5 significantly. Eosinophilia, mucus hypersecretion, and airway hyperresponsiveness were also reduced. Even though they were carried out in different ways, the studies all agree on the scientific evidence that shows that taking resveratrol orally is a good way to treat asthma.

Boswellia

Boswellia is a genus of trees that makes frankincense oil by cutting holes in the trunks of the trees. Polysaccharides, resin, and 30–60% essential oils make up this oil. The Boswellia bio-actives are boswellic acids and AKBA (3-O-acetyl-11-keto-boswellic acid), both of which prevent NF-B activation and, as a result, inhibit IL-1, IL-2, IL-4, IL-6, and IFN-gamma release. Studies conducted with this product evaluated its pharmacological activities. Additionally, they prevent leukotriene release by inhibiting it. As a result, once these enzymes and mediators are involved in asthma-related inflammation, it is possible to infer that these compounds from the tree genus may act as anti-asthma molecules based on the physiopathology of asthma. In addition, Boswellia serrata, Curcuma longa, and Glycyrrhiza were found to have a significant impact on the management of bronchial asthma in another study aimed at assessing these compounds' antiasthma activity indicating their potential as an asthma treatment.

Homemade asthma remedies made from animal products

Asthma-Related Natural Products Derived from Animals Natural products derived from animals continue to make up a small percentage of the natural sources for asthma-related products. Still, a lot of studies say that animal-based products like oils, milk, and spleen can be used as a complement to treat a lot of diseases, like asthma. When they are rich in compounds like lipids, prostaglandins, unsaturated fatty acids, enzymes, and polysaccharides, which are responsible for their pharmacological activities, some animal parts and animal products are said to be beneficial in traditional medicine]. Animal sources are also frequently mentioned as biocompatible and biodegradable, suggesting that they can be used safely. The fact that the substances and products referred to in this session can be obtained from a variety of sources, including mammals, amphibians, and crustaceans, demonstrates the extensive scope of their applications.

Holothuroidea, Penaeus, and Sarcophyton ehrenberg are species of marine animals.

Sea Animal Source: Due to their extensive biodiversity, which includes animals and plants that are unique to this environment, marine ecosystems like Holothuroidea, Penaeus, and Sarcophyton ehrenberg are important sources of natural compounds. Algae and sea animals' potential as antimicrobial, anti-inflammatory, antiviral, and antiasthmatic agents have thus been the subject of numerous studies.

Due to its pharmacological activity in treating hypertension, asthma, rheumatism, cuts, burns, and constipation, the sea cucumber, a marine invertebrate animal that belongs to the class

Holothuroidea and is typically found in benthic areas and deep seas, has been used as an elixir in traditional medicine by Asian and Middle Eastern communities. The presence of saponins, cerebrosides, polysaccharides, and peptides in its composition is responsible for these pharmacological activities. Bordbar and others mentioned an experimental study by Herencia et al. in a review of the literature in which sea cucumber extract reduced the enzymatic activity of cyclooxygenase in inflamed mouse tissues without altering the cyclooxygenase enzyme, demonstrating that sea cucumber extract is an effective natural remedy that can be used to treat a variety of inflammatory conditions

The pharmacological activity of chitin, the primary compound of the shrimp (Penaeus) exoskeleton and a polysaccharide formed by repeated units of N-acetylglucosamine to form a long chain through -(1-4) linkage, was studied by Ozdemir and colleagues. Chitin microparticles were administered intravenously to asthma-induced mice in this study, resulting in a decrease in airway hypersensitivity as well as a decrease in serum IgE and peripheral blood eosinophilia [87]. Another study found and isolated ten new prostaglandin derivatives from Sarcophyton ehrenbergi extract, a soft coral species found in the Red Sea. Five of these derivatives showed inhibitory activity against PDE4 (44.3 percent) at 10 g.mL-1, indicating that they could be used to treat asthma and COPD, as PDE4 is the drug target for both conditions

Lastly, these studies demonstrated the need for additional research into marine sources due to the abundance of bio products and/or bioactive with potential anti-inflammatory and asthmatic properties in this environment.

Bullfrog (Rina Cartesian Shaw) Oil

Oil of the Bullfrog (Rina Cartesian Shaw) Bullfrog oil is a natural oil that is obtained from the adipose tissue of the amphibian Rina Cartesian Shaw. The bullfrog is a native of North America whose meat is widely sold worldwide. Traditional medicine has used this oil to treat inflammatory conditions, particularly asthma. The therapeutic qualities of this oil are composed of a blend of mono- and polyunsaturated fatty acids and a bile-derived steroid molecule (ethyl iso-allocate)

The presence of oleic, linolenic, stearic, palmitic, and myristic fatty acids, according to Yaqoob can facilitate the suppression of immune cell functions [58]. It is possible to infer from this evidence that the chemical composition of bullfrog oil makes it suitable for the treatment of asthma and other conditions associated with inflammation. However, in order to verify this hypothesis, additional research is required.

In a study conducted by Neamati and colleagues the buffalo spleen liquid was examined after pigs were anesthetized with ovalbumin and given the adjuvant based on buffalo spleen liquid. When compared to healthy animals, sensitized animals had a lower number of white blood cells and a lower tracheal response in lung lavage This suggests that this fluid may help control asthma. Based on these reports and historical facts regarding the use of microorganisms as a source for the isolation of new bioactive and the development of medicines, it is important to highlight that these new agents may contribute to the current asthma treatment. The use of bacteria and fungi metabolites to treat several diseases is widely reported since the discovery of penicillin. Another study was conducted to evaluate the anti-asthma activity using milk and colostrums. However, the antiasthmatic properties of these metabolites have been the subject of more recent research In light of this concern, Lu and colleagues evaluated the bacterial lysate OM-85 Broncho-Vaxom (BV), a patented pharmaceutical product,'s anti-asthma activity in a study. This book found that the conventional treatment, when combined with bacterial lysate, was able to increase the rate of natural killer T cells in the peripheral blood, lower the level of cytokines (the type of cytokines has not been specified), and then help alleviate asthma symptoms. In addition, the in vivo anti-inflammatory activity of kefir, a fermented milk beverage made from bacteria's lactic and acetic acids was examined. Kefiran, an insoluble polysaccharide, is the primary component of kefir. INF- and TNF- production as well as the release of IL-4, IL-6, and IL-10 were all reduced at normal levels by this compound

.

Chapter 6

Active Pharmaceutical Components from Natural Sources, Widely Used

Natural products have been widely employed as a complementary therapy for asthma therapy, as was previously shown. Similarly, in a mouse asthma model, the intragastric infusion of kefiran promoted the reduction in cytokine production brought on by OVA. While some study on these items focused on isolating chemicals to create new medications based on natural synthesized pharmaceuticals, other studies examined their efficacy as a matrix of substances to supplement or replace the present asthma treatment.

Natural ingredients have traditionally contributed significantly to the development of drugs that may be purchased to treat a number of disorders. Thanks to the identification and isolation of their bioactive compounds, not only were their therapeutic properties assessed, but also the pharmacophore groups and radicals responsible for their toxicity and biopharmaceutical characteristics were found. This study outlines the experimental research that, over the past ten years, have discovered the chemicals that give many natural sources their anti-asthma properties. On the basis of such research, it is really conceivable to alter the structure or delivery of these compounds in a way that would increase their safety or that would enable them to modulate their half-life, allowing them to be targeted to particular action sites total, these studies provided preliminary information that necessitates additional research on these compounds before they can be used to design medicines shortly. Ipratropium bromide, theophylline, epinephrine, and sodium cromoglycate are just a few natural-based active compounds that are currently on the market

Ipratropium bromide, an anticholinergic medication that can make the airways expand, has been widely used to treat asthma. This compound was made from atropine, which was first extracted from Atropa belladonna L in 1809, but it can also be found in other Solanaceae-family plants. Despite this, its chemical structure was only discovered in 1833, and its clinical application took place in 1850, allowing for a thorough understanding of its in vivo biopharmaceutical and therapeutic properties. Theophylline is a commonly prescribed antiasthmatic medication that promotes bronchodilation and reduces asthma inflammation in patients with severe persistent asthma. This molecule, also known as 1,3-dimethylxanthine, was extracted in 1888 from Theobroma cacao L. and Camellia sinensis L., two widely distributed plants. This medication was first used to treat asthma in 1922. Epinephrine, also known as adrenaline, was extracted from Ephedra sinica, a plant that is used a lot in Chinese traditional medicine. This made it possible to make beta-agonist antiasthmatic drugs like salbutamol and salmeterol, which are used to treat asthma today

Additionally, sodium cromoglycate, a drug made from the khellin bioactive extracted from Ammi visnaga (L) Lamk, has been used as a bronchodilator because it inhibits mast cell degranulation.

In general, these reports emphasize the significance of discovering and isolating novel bioactive compounds with potential antiasthmatic properties. The experimental studies that evaluate the activity of compounds obtained from a variety of natural sources may enable the development of new antiasthmatic medications shortly, as the medications that are currently used to treat asthma have been the subject of extensive research over the past few decades.

The Best Asthma Medication

The Best Asthma Treatment The majority of asthma medications are inhaled and directly reach the lungs to open the airways or reduce chronic inflammation. If your asthma isn't well controlled or if you have allergic asthma, which occurs when you are exposed to allergens, you can also add oral medications and injections to your treatment plan.

However, there is no "best" medication for asthma. Instead, you can choose from a variety of short-term and long-term asthma treatments based on how important they are to your care, how bad your asthma is, and what causes it.

A list of the asthma medications that are currently available is provided below. Talk to your doctor about your asthma symptoms and the frequency with which they occur to determine the best treatment plan and medication for you.

Fast-Acting Inhalers

Quick-Relief Inhalers are short-term medications for acute asthma symptoms like wheezing, chest tightness, shortness of breath, and coughing. Rescue inhalers are another name for them.

All asthma sufferers should have access to a quick-relief inhaler. It could be all that is required for mild asthmatic symptoms. These asthma episodes, which are typically referred to as intermittent asthma, occur twice per week or less, with nighttime symptoms occurring no more than twice per month. asthma brought on by exercise. Physical activity is a trigger for this kind of asthma.

Chapter 7

Home cures and natural asthma treatments

Home remedies can help manage asthma symptoms in addition to prescription medication and a well-thought-out treatment strategy.

The defining feature of asthma is airway inflammation in the lungs. The airways enlarge, become more constricted, produce more mucus, and the muscles around the airways get tighter, making breathing more difficult.

There are over 24 million people with asthma in the United States, and they may have to stay home from work or go to the hospital. The condition occasionally has a fatal outcome.

Asthma sufferers can frequently manage their day-to-day symptoms with home remedies and treatments. However, these should only be used in conjunction with, not in place of, a person's medical treatment plan.

Yoga and self-care phone apps, among other home remedies for asthma symptoms, are discussed in detail in this book

suggest that regular breathing exercises can help people with asthma get rid of their symptoms and improve their overall quality of life.

lowering of tension

Reduce stress and other strong emotions like rage can sometimes cause asthma attacks. Home remedies for asthma may be beneficial if they aid in stress reduction.

If someone doesn't have access to an inhaler when they have an asthma attack, they might find these helpful to try along with breathing exercises.

Some methods that people might find useful are:

During an asthma attack, if a person does not have their inhaler on hand, deep breathing, mindfulness meditation, massage therapy, and hypnotherapy may also be helpful. Knowledge of breathing exercises that reduce hyperventilation may also be helpful.

However, there is insufficient research in the area. Breathing exercises probably do not help alleviate asthma symptoms, according to a 2020 review by Trusted Source. To confirm the efficacy of breathing exercises in alleviating asthma symptoms, additional research is required.

During an asthma attack, the Buteyko method and the Papworth method are two common breathing techniques.

locating and removing triggers

Identifying and eliminating asthma attack triggers Identifying and eliminating asthma attack triggers is one of the most effective home remedies for asthma. Trusted Source: While these may vary from person to person, some common triggers include dust mites, mold, air pollution, cockroaches, respiratory infections like influenza, especially from smoking tobacco, but also from burning wood or grass.

emotional stress and cold air can also exacerbate asthma symptoms in some people, especially if they exercise outside in the cold. However, most of the time, they can exercise without experiencing any symptoms with the assistance of effective treatment and management.

A person who is aware of their asthma triggers can take steps to avoid them. This may include the following:

avoiding smoking and inhaling secondhand smoke, using allergy-proof bedding, washing and drying it weekly, vacuuming frequently, storing food in airtight containers to keep pests out, regularly cleaning the storage and dining areas, and installing an air filter in the bedroom. Taking herbal remedies and supplements Some people may find that various herbal remedies and supplements help alleviate the symptoms of asthma.

Herbal remedies and supplements

However, it is essential to note that herbal remedies and supplements should not be used in place of True Source clinical treatments.

Reviews indicate that taking vitamin D supplements may be beneficial to some individuals. Trusted Source However, there is a lack of agreement regarding the advantages of vitamin D in the treatment of asthma, and research is ongoing.

In a similar vein, a 2018 study found that some formulas of Chinese herbal medicines can alleviate the symptoms of acute asthma. But no other controlled studies have been able to replicate these results.

When considering home remedies for asthma, individuals should exercise caution and talk to a healthcare professional about all aspects of managing the condition. A treatment's popularity does not guarantee its safety or effectiveness.

For instance, some herbal remedies may exacerbate asthma symptoms.

St. John's wort may decrease the effectiveness of theophylline, an asthma relief medication that is frequently prescribed by doctors. As a result, a person's asthma symptoms may get worse.

ButterburTrusted Source-containing unregulated products can also cause serious side effects like damage to the liver.

Chapter 8

Foods That Help and Harm With Asthma and Your Diet

Fruits and vegetables may be helpful.
Foods that can be useful and harmful include: No asthma diet, other than fruits and vegetables, can solve your breathing issues. Certain meals, nevertheless, might be healthy for you. Fruits and vegetables are a fantastic place to start. Vitamins E and C and beta carotene are antioxidants that help stop "free radicals" from causing cellular damage and possibly inflaming and aggravating your lungs.

Might Help: Vitamin D
Comes primarily from sunlight, but it can also be found in some foods. Fatty fish like salmon and swordfish are the best option, followed by milk, eggs, and orange juice, which are often "fortified" with vitamin D. Vitamin D boosts the immune system's response, which is your body's defense

against germs, and may help reduce swelling in your airways. Having low levels of vitamin D can increase the number of asthma attacks.

Seeds and nuts could be helpful

contain a lot of good things, but vitamin E, which is found in raw seeds, almonds, hazelnuts, and cruciferous vegetables like broccoli and kale, may be beneficial for asthma patients. Tocopherol, a chemical found in vitamin E, may reduce asthmatic coughing and wheezing. Research is underway.

Might Hurt: Dried Fruit

Dried fruits are one of the foods you should probably avoid if you have asthma. Although fresh fruit, particularly oranges, and apples, can assist in asthma control, the sulfites that help preserve dried fruit may exacerbate some people's asthma. Sulfites can also be found in shrimp, pickled vegetables, maraschino cherries, bottled lemon juice, and alcohol, particularly red wine.

Might Hurt: Beans

It all comes down to how much gas they give some people. It can make it harder to breathe and bloat your belly. Even worse, it might set off an asthma attack. The most well-known candidate is beans. To lessen this effect, soak them for a few hours and change the water a few times. Garlic, onions, fried foods, carbonated drinks, and other foods can also cause gas.

May Hurt: Coffee

Salicylates in coffee are chemicals that are naturally found in coffee, tea, herbs, spices, and even aspirin, an anti-inflammatory medication. Even though most people don't react to them, if you already have asthma, they could make it harder to breathe. If you eliminate as many of these from your diet as you can, you might be able to alleviate these symptoms.

The Mediterranean diet may be useful.

Might Help: Whole grains, beans, nuts, and a lot of fruits and vegetables are included in the Mediterranean diet. You limit your consumption of red meat and eat fish and chicken at least twice per week. Olive or canola oil is used in cooking, and herbs are used as a flavoring instead of salt. Even some red wine is available as an option for adults. According to some studies, people who eat this way may have fewer attacks of asthma and have a lower risk of developing the condition in the first place. More research is required.

May Help: Fish/Omega-3

Might Help: Fish The omega-3 fatty acids, particularly those found in fatty fish like salmon, herring, tuna, and sardines, are everything. They assist in reducing your body's production of IgE. That is an antibody that can make asthmatics' breathing difficult. However, the high oral steroid doses that some people need to take to treat very serious asthma can prevent much of this beneficial effect from happening.

May Hurt: Food Allergies

Might Hurt: Food Allergies If you have asthma, you are more likely to have a food allergy. Additionally, wheezing and other asthma symptoms may result from a food reaction. If you exercise after eating certain foods, it may make things worse in some cases. Try to notice what causes it and stay away from it. Even though each person is unique, common triggers include shellfish, nuts, dairy, and wheat.

May Hurt: Too Much Food

Your body stores extra calories in fat cells when you consume more calories than you burn. If you do that too much, you might start to put on weight. If your body mass index (BMI) is 30 or higher, you are more likely to develop asthma and your symptoms may get worse. Additionally, you might not respond as well to standard treatments like asthma attack-stopping inhaled steroids.

May Help: Tomatoes

Might Help: Tomatoes It appears that asthmatics benefit from eating foods made with tomatoes. Although more research is required, scientists believe that lycopene may be the most beneficial component. They have been shown to improve breathing over time, according to some studies. Who wants marinara pasta?

May Help: Variety

Might Help: Variety no one food is a "magic bullet" that will cure asthma. To keep your body healthy enough to handle attacks when they happen or prevent them altogether, you need a variety of vitamins and nutrients. Any significant dietary changes you make should be discussed with your doctor because they may have an impact on your condition and your medication.

May Hurt: Supplements

Might Hurt: Supplements As a general rule, food-based nutrients work better to prevent asthma than supplements do. Get your vegetables, then! Also, nuts. also, fish and produce). You might have heard that particular "soy is flavone" supplements can alleviate asthma symptoms. This may be the case for some asthmatics, according to some studies, but more research is needed.

May Hurt: Liquid Nitrogen

Liquid Nitrogen There are various names for it, but some people refer to it as a "nitro puff." A fancy cocktail, a brand-new frozen dessert at the mall, or other foods might produce a smoky, icy stream. It may appear to be fun, but it's best not to do it. It could also seriously harm your skin and even internal organs, which is especially dangerous if you have asthma.

Workout Safely Despite Severe Asthma

Exercise Safely If You Have Severe Asthma Yes, You Can Work Out 1/14 It can help you stay in shape. You should be able to participate in the majority of types of exercise as long as your asthma is under control. If you want to get the most out of your workouts and stay safe in the event of an attack while you're at the gym, follow these guidelines.

Go Cardio

Anything that makes your heart beat faster, such as swimming, biking, walking, or jogging, can help. Maintain a low level of activity. What is that implying? While you're doing it, you should be able to talk. Be familiar with your body and asthma, as well as your triggers. While the circumstances surrounding exercise may be problematic, exercise itself may not be.

both weight training and yoga

Both yoga and weight lifting help build muscle and get rid of a common asthma trigger: stress. Maintain a moderate level of effort. A good goal for weightlifting is 10 to 15 repetitions. When lifting weights or holding poses, don't hold your breath.

Avoid Pollen

Avoid Pollen If there is a lot of pollen in the air, the great outdoors is not good for asthma. Pollen counts and air quality can both be found in the weather report. Go to the gym instead if it isn't good. Do you suffer from hay fever-like seasonal allergies? Ensure that you also take your allergy medications.

Avoid Pollution

Avoid areas near factories and busy roads. Head indoors if it is cloudy or the air quality report is poor. However, ensure that the air inside is also clean. Asthma can be triggered by dust, cigarette smoke, and pet dander.

Warm Up and Cool Down

Warm-up and cool-down: To get your body ready for exercise, start slowly and stretch your muscles. Slow down and stretch again as you finish. Warm-up and cooling off should take 10 minutes each. Avoid abrupt stops Guard Against the Cold Cold air can cause asthma. Cover your mouth and nose with a scarf if you exercise outside in the cold. It will assist in warming the air before reaching your lungs. Is it ill or rundown? Take a Day Off When you have a cold, the flu, or another illness, you shouldn't exercise. If you exercise while you are ill, you are more likely to have an attack.

The year 2021 marks the 51st anniversary of the Clean Air Act, which was enacted to improve air quality. However, the American Lung Association's annual State of the Air rankings shows that many U.S. cities still have unhealthy levels of smog more than 50 years later. Ozone levels rise as a result of warming caused by climate change, and frequent wildfires worsen air quality.

Chapter 9

Foods That Trigger Asthma Attacks

Your asthma symptoms won't miraculously disappear if you eat particular foods. But your diet can have an effect. Some may even make your asthma symptoms worse. Naturally, not everyone will respond to the same meals in the same manner, but monitoring your response to particular foods and, if necessary, avoiding them, may be beneficial.

1. Sulfites, one of the food additives that many asthmatics find to be the most problematic, are a type of preservative found in dried fruit that is used to increase the food's shelf life. Sulfites are present in many varieties of dried fruit. Look for phrases like "potassium bisulfite" and "sodium sulfite" on the label to see whether those dried cherries or apricots can aggravate your asthma.

2. Sulfites are also present in a lot of wine and beer varieties. If you end up coughing or wheezing after having that glass of cabernet, you might have to give it up. Wine's histamines, according to some research, may also cause symptoms like watery eyes, sneezing, and wheezing

3. Shrimp Consuming shrimp that has been frozen or prepared could pose a risk to you. You are correct if you think that sulfites are to blame once more! Sulfites are a common ingredient in frozen shrimp and other seafood because they prevent the development of unappetizing black spots. Make sure you don't accidentally eat something that has been cooked in a broth made with shrimp or other

4 when you eat out. Pickles The pickle that came with your deli sandwich might need to be tossed. Sulfites are a common preservative in fermented foods like sauerkraut and pickled foods. For the same reason, avoid relishes, horseradish sauce, and even salad dressing mixes.

5. Prepared or packaged potatoes The next time you're tempted to use a mix to make mashed potatoes, think twice. Examine the package's list of ingredients. Potatoes, possibly some vegetable oil, salt, whey powder, or dried nonfat milk are all in that package, but further, down the list, you might find a preservative like sodium bisulfite. The sulfites once more strike! Instead, go with a whole potato that can be baked. Make sure to first poke it a few times with a fork.

6. Maraschino cherries They look like brightly colored jewels in a glass jar, but if you have asthma or are sensitive to sulfites, you should just admire them from a distance. Preservatives that could cause bronchospasms or other asthma symptoms may also be found in fruit juices that are bottled or canned, like lemon and lime juice.

7. Anything to which you are allergic You probably already know to be on the lookout for foods that you are allergic to. Keep up the good work, as those foods may also contribute to asthma attacks. According to the American Academy of Allergy, Asthma, and Immunology, cow's milk, tree nuts, wheat, soy, peanuts, eggs, fish, and shellfish account for the majority of allergic reactions. Avoid eating them or anything that is cross-contaminated with them if you are allergic to any of them.

Adapting Your Lifestyle Can Reduce Asthma Attacks

The Centers for Disease Control and Prevention (CDC) estimates that approximately 6 million children under the age of 18 in the United States suffer from asthma. The frequency of attacks can be decreased by making lifestyle changes. Asthma is a condition that can be managed, but it can also be fatal. There is no known cure for asthma, which accounts for nine deaths per day. However, living with asthma need not be frightening for either you or your child. Your child's condition can be managed and the likelihood of an attack can be reduced.

Understanding the difference between asthma attacks and chronic asthma Asthma affects the lungs and airways. Exercise-induced asthma, allergic asthma, and nocturnal asthma are the most prevalent types of asthma.

Asthmatic individuals frequently have inflamed bronchial tubes, making them extremely sensitive to environmental triggers like pollen, pet dander, noxious fumes, and a wide variety of other substances.

Asthma typically presents with chest tightness, shortness of breath, wheezing or whistling while breathing, and coughing, particularly in the early morning or at night. An asthma attack is indicated when these symptoms become severe and breathing becomes more difficult.

Things you can do to keep asthma under control: Understanding the disease and making a few changes to your lifestyle can help your child manage their asthma and reduce their attacks.

If your child has asthma, the first thing you should do is figure out what sets off their attacks. You need to be aware of your child's triggers to assist them in avoiding them because everyone has different triggers. Secondhand smoke, perfumes, and other odors that can cause an attack are all potential irritants to the lungs.

Invest in a HEPA filter If your child suffers from allergic asthma, a HEPA filter might be a good investment. While filtering the air in your home, high-efficiency particulate air (HEPA) filters catch irritants. Houseplants that purify the air are another option if you're on a tight budget because these filters can be pricey.

Maintain a clean home while exercising caution when using cleaning products. Keep up with your cleaning so that your home is as free of mold and dust as possible. Because harsh chemicals can irritate your child's lungs and airways, you might also want to consider switching to chemical-free cleaning products.

Maintaining a healthy weight and fitness level is beneficial for your child's overall health, but it is especially important for children with chronic conditions like asthma. Eat healthy and exercise (with caution). Your child's symptoms and attacks may get worse if they are overweight or don't get enough exercises

Additionally, avoid giving your asthmatic child dairy products because they produce mucus and can cause attacks. To avoid the ingredients that cause your child's attacks, be aware of how certain foods affect them and prioritize home-cooked meals.

Create a plan of action Create an asthma action plan for your child and educate friends, family, and teachers about it. By doing this, you can rest assured that everyone in your child's life is aware of the medications that are required and how to spot an approaching attack. Included in this strategy ought to be ensuring that your child always has their inhaler on hand.

You need a specialist who will be there for your child if they have asthma. Your specialist is waiting. Margaret Lubega, MD, and her trusted team of specialists at First Pediatric Care Center are here for your child and the rest of your family.

We offer a full range of pediatric services, including sick visits on the same day, for infants through young adults. Our No. 1 priority is patient care and long-term relationships. Priority one. Call or make an appointment online right away if you want an experienced and trustworthy specialist to take care of your family's needs.

Other Products Derived from Animals even though the majority of the animal products that are currently used in traditional medicine to treat asthma are derived from animal tissues, there is evidence that mammal fluids, such as buffalo spleen liquid, milk, and colostrum, can influence the immune system and help alleviate asthma symptoms.

Conclusion

While asthma can be managed, it cannot be cured. You and your doctor must create a personalized asthma treatment plan for you because everyone has a different type of asthma. Your plan will contain an asthma action plan with details on your triggers and directions for administering your meds.

Your airways become smaller or narrower due to swelling in the airways, excessive mucus that obstructs the airways, and muscles that tighten and squeeze around the airways. This makes it harder for air to move past your airways, which makes breathing more challenging. Asthma medicines can address these three alterations. They widen your airways and facilitate breathing.